Table of Contents

How much sugar per day do Americans consume? According to research done by the U.S. Department of Agriculture, although Americans appear to be consuming less sugar today than in the previous couple of decades, average sugar consumption in America is still around 94 grams per day, or 358 calories. That's a lot of sugar, but it doesn't have to be this way. In fact, you can even follow a sugar-free diet to help lower this number greatly.

A great deal of research has shown that removing sources of excess sugar from your diet not only helps with weight loss, but can also reduce your risk for common health problems like type 2 diabetes, digestive problems, autoimmune conditions and more. Cutting out sugar is a great way to detox your body because sugar is bad for you. So, what can you eat that has no sugar in it but is still satisfying?

Proteins — like grass-fed meat, eggs or fish, for example — lots of veggies, healthy fats, nuts, seeds and other detoxifying foods are where you'll get the bulk of your calories when eating a low-sugar or sugar-free diet. While the transition away from eating lots of sugar might seem hard at first, provoking cravings and even other symptoms that can mimic a "withdrawal," within a few weeks you'll likely see your efforts start to pay off.

High sugar consumption can increase inflammation, mess with hormone production, rob you of energy, and even interfere with your mood and sleep. That's why kicking your sugar addiction, replacing "empty"calories with nutrient-dense ones, will noticeably change you how you feel, both mentally and physically, in many ways.

Chapter one

What Is a Sugar-Free Diet?

A sugar-free diet (or no-sugar diet) is one that typically limits all sources of added sugar (like soda, snack bars and desserts, for example) and hidden sugar foods, and it sometimes also encourages a reduction in high-carbohydrate foods (like grains or fruits) that can still be healthy but do contain natural sugars.

There isn't just one way to eat a low-sugar diet, but rather a variety of different plans depending on your goals and preferences. You might choose to eliminate basically all sources of sugar from your diet, including things like fruit and even some veggies, or to only eliminate sweetened processed foods that are high in empty calories.

Either way, there are lots of benefits to consuming more satisfying, nourishing foods in sugar's place, such as lean proteins and healthy fats. Another perk is that most low-sugar or sugar-free diets don't require calorie counting, since eliminating processed foods is usually enough to produce results on its own.

Some of the benefits of reducing your sugar intake in place of eating more whole foods include:

- Help with losing weight and preventing obesity
- Lowered risk for type 2 diabetes or prediabetes
- Gaining more energy
- Having more stabile moods
- Reduced risk for inflammatory digestive conditions, such as irritable bowel disease (IBD), Crohn's disease, candida, IBS and intolerance to wheat/gluten or FODMAP foods — many also notice less constipation, diarrhea, stomach bloating or acid reflux
- When sugar contributes to obesity, a sugar-free diet lowers risk for conditions related to metabolic syndrome, such atherosclerosis, hypertension and heart disease
- Possibly less risk for cancer

- Protection against fatty liver disease
- Better protection against other common conditions related to inflammation, weight gain and nutrient deficiencies like hemorrhoids, kidney stones, peptic ulcer, PMS, autoimmune diseases, polycystic ovarian syndrome, and neurological diseases like dementia or Alzheimer's disease
- In order to reduce your sugar intake and deal with cravings for sweets or refined carbohydrates — a very common problem among most people looking to lose weight or improve their eating habits — there are five main steps I recommend taking, which are discussed in more detail below:
- Eat more fiber.
- Include more protein in your diet.
- Eat more healthy fats.
- Consume sour (including probiotic/fermented) foods.
- Read ingredient labels carefully when grocery shopping in order to know just what you're consuming, since most people don't realize how much sugar they're really eating or drinking.

Why is a high-sugar diet bad for you? Sugar can change the gut microbiota in a way that increases intestinal permeability, increasing inflammation. It can also contribute to overeating and obesity, causing many negative changes in the body.

Eating a low-sugar, low-glycemic index diet can help balance your blood sugar levels throughout the day, prevent insulin resistance (one long-term effect of a high-sugar diet), protect you from fatty liver disease and heart disease, control your appetite, and keep you fuller and energized for longer.

A low-sugar or sugar-free diet is very similar to what's called a "low-glycemic index diet." The definition of the glycemic index (GI) is "a measure of the blood glucose-raising potential of the carbohydrate content of a food, compared to a reference food (generally pure glucose, or sugar)." A food's GI number tells you how quickly the food is converted into sugar once you eat it; the higher the GI number, the more drastically the food will cause your blood sugar level to increase.

All carbohydrates increase blood glucose (sugar), but this doesn't mean that all carbohydrates are necessarily unhealthy and should be avoided. Sugary, processed foods impact blood glucose levels a lot more than whole, unprocessed foods. For example, table sugar, white bread, white rice, white potatoes, white flour and all other types of sweeteners have high GI values.

Factors that determine a food's GI value include how much sugar the food contains, how processed it is, the fiber content and what other types of foods it's paired with (this determines "the glycemic load").

The types of high-GI foods that contain lots of added sugar and/or refined grains that you should remove from your diet include:

- refined grain products made with white flours
- most breads, processed breakfast cereals, cookies, snack bars, cakes, desserts, etc.
- sweetened dairy products
- sweetened beverages, such as soda and bottled juices
- all types of table/cane sugar

Sometimes all other natural sweeteners should be excluded, too, depending on the state of your health, like honey, syrups, molasses, etc., and in some cases, other sweet ingredients like dried fruits (raisins, craisins and dates) and starchy root vegetables (like white potatoes, beets or winter squash) need to be limited in order to see results.

How does a sugar-free diet compare to the ketogenic diet and other low-carb diets?

If you exclude all sources of sugar from your diet, you're already on your way to eating a low-carb diet, since sugary foods provide the body with high amounts of glucose. Once glucose supply is reduced, the body burns fat for fuel instead of glucose from carbohydrates or sugar.

When sugar is taken out of the equation, your carb intake then depends on how many grains, veggies, legumes and other sources of carbs you still eat in proportion to fats and protein.

The keto diet is a very low-carb diet that includes virtually no sugar and only about 20–50 grams of net carbs daily. The majority of calories on the keto diet come from fats, like coconut oil, butter or fattier cuts of meat. Sugary, high-carb foods are eliminated, including grains, fruit, dairy and beans.

A sugar-free diet is one type of low-carb diet plan, among many different variations. How many carbs are typically in a low-carb diet? It depends a lot on the individual plan being followed, but most moderate plans range from about 50–130 grams of net carbs daily. Usually the lower the carb intake, the faster that weight loss will happen. However, a very low-carb diet isn't always sustainable for some people or realistic, so a moderate low-carb plan may be a better fit.

Best Sugar-Free Foods

Healthy protein foods

Grass-fed beef, lamb, venison or other game

Free-range poultry like chicken or turkey

High-quality protein powders, including bone broth, collagen, whey protein (ideally from raw goat milk) or pea protein

Lentils, beans and other legumes (ideally soaked and sprouted to help with digestion)

Wild fish like salmon, mackerel, tuna, etc.

Organic natto or tempeh (fermented soybean product)

Raw milk and fermented dairy products like kefir or yogurt

Free-range eggs

Raw cheese

High-fiber foods (may contain small amounts of natural sugars)

Cruciferous veggies like cabbage, broccoli, Brussels sprouts, etc.

Other veggies (aim for a combination of cooked and raw) like bell peppers, cucumber, carrots, green peas, okra, turnips, squash, zucchini, asparagus, tomatoes, mushrooms, artichokes, etc.

Chia seeds and flaxseeds

Avocados

Coconut flakes

Berries

Beans like black beans, navy beans, adzuki, lentils, lima, split, mung, etc.

In moderate amounts, whole grains like quinoa, brown rice, oats, amaranth, buckwheat, teff, farro, etc.

In smaller amounts, other fruits that are a bit higher in sugar, like apples, bears, figs, prunes, oranges, grapefruit, melon or kiwi

Healthy fats

Coconut oil, milk, butter or cream

Real virgin olive oil

Grass-fed butter

Nuts like walnuts, almonds, cashews, Brazil nuts, etc.

Seeds like chia, flax, pumpkin, sunflower, etc.

Avocado

Other oils like MCT oil, palm fruit oil, hemp seed, flaxseed, avocado oil, etc.

Sour foods, probiotic foods and other detoxifying ingredients

Cultured veggies like salted gherkin pickles, olives or kimchi

Kombucha or coconut kefir

Natto, tempeh or miso

Kvass

Raw cheese

Lemon and lime juice

Apple cider vinegar (use some in salad dressing or in water with some lemon juice)

Bone broth

All fresh herbs and spices, like ginger, garlic, parsley, oregano, turmeric, etc.

Stevia (extract, green crystalized or drops). Stevia is a no-calorie, natural sweetener that makes a good sugar substitute in recipes. Use it in drinks or on foods in place of regular white table sugar.

Diet Plan

Read ingredient labels carefully so you know exactly what's in the food you consume. This is especially important when buying or using "sneaky" sugary foods like condiments, sauces, canned foods, beverages, etc.

To keep your appetite in check, aim to get about 35–40 grams of fiber per day. Start by consuming more high-fiber foods like fresh vegetables and nuts and seeds, such as chia seeds and flaxseeds.

Drink enough water to help with digestion and elimination. Aim to have about eight glasses per day.

If you do need to sweeten foods, try stevia first (rather than artificial sweeteners). If you can't stand the taste of stevia, in small amounts you may want to use some natural sweeteners from time to time, such as raw honey, blackstrap molasses, dates or pureed fruit (like bananas or apples).

Also avoid too much caffeine or alcohol. Many mixed drinks tend to be high in sugar and calories, plus alcohol can spike your appetite and cause cravings.

Even if the food is low in sugar/carbs, try to limit packaged foods from your diet that are highly processed and very salty. Additionally, replace fast foods and fried foods with healthier options you can cook at home — this way you can control the ingredients.

Avoid eating foods with the following types/names of sugar and sweeteners: white granulated sugar, dextrose, fructose, brown sugar, confectioner's powdered sugar, corn syrup and high-fructose corn syrup, invert sugar, lactose, malt syrup, maltose, molasses, nectars (for example, peach or pear nectar), raw sugar, sucrose and others.

Aim to eat balanced meals that include a healthy source of protein, some veggies and some healthy fat. This combination will help keep you more satisfied, energized and focused throughout the day. If you include some carbohydrates, try to make it a complex carb that has some fiber, and keep an eye on your portion sizes.

Don't drink your calories. Avoid soda, juice or artificially sweetened drinks. Instead of adding sugar to beverages, try consuming plain water, seltzer, herbal tea, bone broth or black coffee. In moderate amounts, unsweetened coconut milk or water can also be a good choice.

Sugar-free meal ideas

For breakfast — unsweetened oats with nuts, seeds, coconut milk, stevia and cinnamon; avocado toast with hard boiled eggs; unsweetened goat's milk yogurt with grain-free granola; a homemade green smoothie.

For lunch — a large salad with sliced chicken and avocado; some quiche with soup and a salad; a salmon or turkey burger; homemade brown rice bowl with veggies and beans.

For dinner — a palm-sized serving of steak with veggies, and possibly some rice or quinoa; a piece of fish with salad, veggies and half a sweet potato; a burrito, tacos or empanadas made with chorizo and veggies; balsamic chicken with tomato and mozzarella; brown rice, broccoli and chicken stir-fry.

What Natural Sugars Are Necessary for Health?

If you're looking to start a low-carb or sugar-free diet, you may be wondering if you'll still eat enough "healthy carbohydrates" to keep your body functioning properly. While it's true that we all need at least some carbohydrates in order to fuel physical activity, repair damaged tissue, and supply our bodies and brains with energy, the amount we need is less than most people typically consume.

Here are some of the reasons that you'll want to keep at least some carbohydrates in your diet, which may include some natural sugars found in things like fruits or veggies:

Plant-based foods that contain carbohydrates, and sometimes natural sugars, also provider dietary fiber. Fiber does not actually get fully digested once consumed, which is why people following a low-carb diet usually don't count grams of fiber toward their net carb intake. Net carbs are the grams of carbs left over when grams of fiber are subtracted from the total amount.

Fiber is needed for digestive health, cardiovascular health and controlling appetite hormones.

Fiber is also typically found in low-calorie foods that are high in vitamins, minerals and antioxidants. For example, high-fiber foods include leafy green veggies, berries, apples, beans, seeds avocados and sweet potatoes. Not all of these foods are "sugar-free," but the sugar they do contain is naturally occurring and often not a problem considering all the other nutrients available in the food.

The whole foods described above are low in calories but good sources of electrolytes, like potassium and magnesium, as well as antioxidants like carotenoids, beta-carotene, lycopene, vitamin E and vitamin C.

Compared to a sugar-free diet, what foods would be included in a grain-free or wheat-free diet?

A grain-free diet/gluten-free diet eliminates all grains, especially wheat, but this doesn't mean it's necessarily low in sugar. Gluten is a protein found in wheat, barley and rye. A gluten-free diet, therefore, removes all sources of these grains, including most baked goods, bread, rolls, desserts, cereal, etc.

A grain-free diet takes things a step further and also removes ALL other grains, like quinoa, oats, buckwheat, etc. If sugar is also removed from these diets, then it's basically the same thing as eating a low-carb diet.

Side Effects

Depending on how many carbohydrates you continue to consume once cutting out sugar, you may notice some side effects when changing your diet. Usually these will go away within one to three weeks as your body gets used to eating less processed foods and consuming more healthy fats and fiber.

You may want to transition into a lower-carb, sugar-free diet gradually in order to help your digestive system and appetite adjust. While altering your diet, it isn't unusual to temporarily experience some of the following side effects:

- Low energy or fatigue
- Digestive issues like bloating or gassiness
- Cravings
- Brain fog
- Changes in your sleep and appetite

How to do a No-Sugar Diet Works

To maintain a healthy perspective on sugar consumption, it's essential to consider the guidelines set forth by the American Heart Association (AHA), which include the following:

For men, the recommended daily limit of added sugar is no more than 9 teaspoons, equivalent to 36 grams (g) or 150 calories.

Women should aim for an even lower threshold, limiting their added sugar intake to 6 teaspoons, which translates to 25 g or 100 calories per day.

For context, a single 12-ounce can of soda contains 8 teaspoons of sugar, amounting to 32 g of added sugar.

The AHA recommends limiting added sugars to 6% or fewer of your daily caloric intake.4 The U.S. Department of Agriculture's (USDA) 2020–2025 Dietary Guidelines for Americans advises restricting the consumption of added sugars to a level that constitutes less than 10% of one's daily calorie intake.

Added sugars are commonly present in items such as:

- Sugary drinks (soft drinks, fruit juice, energy drinks)
- Processed snacks
- Candy
- Desserts made from refined grains
- Canned fruits in syrup
- Baked good
- Energy bars
- Sweetened yogurts
- Sugary breakfast cereals
- Canned or packaged foods

It is important to distinguish that sugars naturally occurring in foods such as fruits and dairy products are not classified as added sugars under these recommendations.

Examples of nutrient-dense foods with no added sugars include:

- Vegetables
- Whole grains
- Seafood
- Eggs
- Legumes (such as beans and lentils)
- Unsalted nuts and seeds
- Dairy products
- Lean cuts of meat and poultry

The AHA and the USDA emphasize the importance of minimizing sugar and eating nutrient-rich foods and drinks that offer valuable vitamins, minerals, and other health-enhancing elements while maintaining low added sugars.

Duration

The duration of a no- or low-sugar diet depends on factors such as your current health status, your weight-management goals, and any underlying medical conditions.

It's important to note that while a no-sugar or low-sugar diet may offer various health benefits, it's essential to consult with a healthcare provider or registered dietitian before making significant dietary changes to ensure it aligns with your individual health goals and needs.

Some people may choose to follow a no- or low-sugar diet for a short time, such as a few weeks or a month. Others may adopt a no- or low-sugar diet as a long-term lifestyle choice. This type of diet can be especially important for individuals with diabetes, insulin resistance (when cells don't respond well to insulin and can't take up glucose from the blood), or obesity, in which managing sugar intake is crucial for overall health.

What to Eat: 7-Day Plan

If you are starting a no- or low-sugar diet, it may help to plan your meals for a week. It is crucial to prioritize the consumption of a diverse array of fruits and vegetables.6 It also means opting for whole grains as the foundation of your grain intake and favoring protein sources that are predominantly plant-based, such as legumes and nuts, alongside fish and seafood.

Here's a sample seven-day meal plan focused on whole, unprocessed foods. It includes various nutrient-rich options aligning with the AHA and USDA guidelines with low or no added sugars. Talk to your healthcare provider or dietician before starting a new diet plan to make sure it is healthy for you.

Day 1

Breakfast: Scrambled eggs with spinach and tomatoes, with a small serving of plain Greek yogurt with a handful of fresh berries

Lunch: Grilled chicken breast with a side salad (lettuce, cucumber, and bell peppers) dressed with olive oil and vinegar

Dinner: Baked salmon with steamed broccoli and quinoa

Day 2

Breakfast: Oatmeal made with rolled oats, unsweetened almond milk, and sliced almonds, with a sprinkle of cinnamon and a few slices of fresh apple (keep the portion small)

Lunch: Turkey and avocado lettuce wraps with a side of carrot and celery sticks

Dinner: Tofu stir-fry with mixed vegetables (broccoli, bell peppers, and snap peas) in a low-sodium soy sauce

Day 3

Breakfast: Cottage cheese with sliced peaches (in moderation) and a sprinkle of chopped nuts

Lunch: Lentil and vegetable soup

Dinner: Grilled shrimp with a side of roasted Brussels sprouts and brown rice

Day 4

Breakfast: Smoothie with unsweetened almond milk, spinach, a scoop of protein powder, and a small amount of berries

Lunch: Quinoa salad with chickpeas, diced cucumber, and a lemon-tahini dressing

Dinner: Baked chicken thighs with asparagus and mashed cauliflower

Day 5

Breakfast: Scrambled eggs with sautéed mushrooms and a side of sliced avocado with whole grain toast

Lunch: Spinach and kale salad with grilled chicken, cherry tomatoes, and a vinaigrette dressing

Dinner: Baked cod with roasted sweet potatoes and steamed green beans

Day 6

Breakfast: Full-fat plain yogurt with chia seeds and a few raspberries

Lunch: Zucchini noodles (zoodles) with pesto sauce and grilled shrimp

Dinner: Beef and vegetable stir-fry with a homemade, low-sugar stir-fry sauce

Day 7

Breakfast: Sliced turkey breast wrapped around avocado slices

Lunch: Cabbage and carrot slaw with grilled salmon and a light vinaigrette dressing

Dinner: Baked chicken breast with a side of roasted mixed vegetables (zucchini, bell peppers, and red onion) and quinoa

For snacks, consider options like raw nuts, celery sticks with almond butter, or cucumber slices with hummus. Always check food labels for hidden sugars, and try to minimize processed foods as much as possible.

More tips to Cut Down on Sugar

Consuming a no- or low-sugar diet may be easier with some of the following tips:

- Eliminate table sugar, syrup, honey, and molasses from your kitchen.
- Reduce sugar in cereal and coffee.
- Replace soda with water or diet drinks.
- Opt for fresh, frozen, or canned fruits.
- Choose fruits in water, not syrup.

- Reduce sugar in baking recipes.
- Use extracts (vanilla, almond) instead.
- Spice up foods without sugar.
- Swap with unsweetened applesauce.

Practical and Realistic

Many diets, particularly those touting weight-loss claims, are not always realistic in practice. Some diets make bold claims of rapid weight loss in a short time. But more often than not, these plans end up backfiring and any weight loss experienced is likely to be regained once regular eating habits are resumed.

A no sugar diet that focuses on whole foods teaches healthy lifestyle habits since cutting out added sugar means you're also cutting out many packaged, processed foods containing artificial ingredients. It is a practical lifestyle to adhere to for not just weight loss but long-term weight management and overall health.

Simple to Follow

A no sugar diet does not have any timelines, guidelines, rules, or restrictions (aside from cutting out added sugars). There are no books to buy (unless you want to learn more) or products or supplements to subscribe to, nor is it promoted by a single celebrity or public figure. All you have to do is eliminate added sugar by eating whole, unprocessed foods whenever possible, making this an easy-to-follow plan.

Flexible and Adaptable

Because there are no hard-and-fast rules on a no sugar diet, what you eat is up to your personal preferences and budget, and the plan is adaptable to suit your lifestyle. In addition, as you slowly wean yourself off sugar and your body starts to naturally crave more nutritious foods, a no sugar diet can encourage mindful, intuitive eating. In time, adhering to the no sugar lifestyle can become second nature rather than a temporary fix or short-term diet.

Long-Term Sustainability

It's healthy and safe to eat this way indefinitely, and sugar cravings should fade over time. As long as you stick with whole foods and read labels carefully, you may find it easy to stick to the no sugar diet for the long term.

Following a no sugar diet (or even a low sugar diet) should offer health benefits including weight loss. But it can be difficult to fully cut added sugar from your diet.

No Guidelines to Follow

Since it's not a formal plan, a no sugar diet has few guidelines other than cutting out added sugars as completely as possible. No calorie- or carb-counting here, or even recommendations for portion control. While this can benefit anyone seeking a less regimented eating plan, some people may need more structure and parameters to meet their weight loss and health goals. For instance, without any calorie requirements to meet, it's still possible to overeat on this plan.

Challenging

Setting aside the common American taste for sugar, there is sugar hiding in many foods (some of them quite unexpected). Distinguishing added sugars from natural sugars can be challenging. As a rule of thumb, your best bet is to stick with real, whole foods and limit many packaged convenience foods. Always read labels carefully to look for added sugars.

Time-Consuming

While following a no-sugar lifestyle is undeniably healthy, keep in mind that you will have to do a lot more meal prep, planning, and cooking. For those who may not have that kind of time, a no sugar diet may not be the most realistic choice.

Is a No Sugar Diet Healthy for You?

Many low-carb eating plans also limit sugar, so those programs can resemble a no sugar diet. Cutting sugar also aligns with government advice on healthy eating. The USDA's dietary guidelines suggest a balanced mix of fruits, grains, vegetables, protein, and dairy products. There's no space for added sugars, but they're also not strictly prohibited.

If weight loss is one of your goals, you may need to count calories in addition to cutting back on added sugars. Avoiding those sugars will likely result in consuming fewer calories altogether, but to know for sure, use this tool to calculate a daily calorie goal, and then an app or journal to track your progress in meeting that goal.

Chapter two

Sugar free diet recipes

Fluffy Microwave Scrambled Eggs

Use your microwave to make light and fluffy scrambled eggs for a quick and easy breakfast to start your day. Follow the technique in this recipe for perfect results every time.

Prep Time: 5 mins

Cook Time: 5 mins

Total Time: 10 mins

Servings: 2

Yield: 2 servings

Microwave Egg Variations

We think this three-ingredient recipe is perfect as it is. But, if you want to dress them up a bit, try one (or more) of these tasty mix-ins:

Cheese

Stir in some shredded Cheddar or Monterey Jack for a cheesy twist.

Ham or Bacon

Diced ham or chopped bacon makes this hearty recipe even more filling.

Veggies

Diced bell peppers, onions, and spinach add color and flavor. To turn up the heat, try jalapeños.

Herbs

Fresh herbs – such as basil, rosemary, oregano, and thyme – lend bright, earthy flavor.

What to Serve With Scrambled Eggs

For a classic breakfast, try pairing these microwave scrambled eggs with Basic Biscuits and Oven-Baked Bacon. You could also make a satisfying Scrambled Egg Sandwich or Breakfast Burrito. With this recipe, it's easy to keep it basic or get as creative as you want. The world is your oyster!

Ingredients

4 eggs

¼ cup milk

⅛ teaspoon salt

Directions

Gather all ingredients.

Break the eggs into a microwave-proof mixing bowl. Add milk and salt; mix well.

Added milk.

Pop the bowl into the microwave and cook on high power for 30 seconds. Remove bowl, beat eggs very well, scraping down the sides of the bowl, and return to the microwave for another 30 seconds.

Repeat this pattern, stirring every 30 seconds for up to 2 1/2 minutes. Stop when eggs have the consistency you desire.

Serve warm and enjoy!

Nutrition Facts (per serving)

141 Calories 9g Fat 2g Carbs 12g Protein

Oven Scrambled Eggs

These baked scrambled eggs are light and fluffy and are a snap to put together for a big crowd. I usually make two pans for our Christmas brunch, and I never have many leftovers!

Prep Time: 10 mins

Cook Time: 20 mins

Total Time: 30 mins

Servings: 12

Yield: 1 9x13-inch dish

Ingredients

½ cup butter or margarine, melted

24 eggs

2 ¼ teaspoons salt

2 ½ cups milk

Directions

Gather all ingredients. Preheat the oven to 350 degrees F (175 degrees C).

Pour melted butter into a 9x13-inch glass baking dish.

Whisk together eggs and salt in a large bowl until well-blended. Gradually whisk in milk. Pour egg mixture into the buttered dish.

Bake uncovered in the preheated oven for 10 to 15 minutes. Stir egg mixture and continue to bake until eggs are set, 10 to 15 minutes more.

Serve and enjoy!

Nutrition Facts (per serving)

236 Calories 19g Fat 3g Carbs 14g Protein

Extreme Veggie Scrambled Eggs

A variety of veggies combined with eggs make a great start to the day.

Prep Time: 10 mins

Cook Time: 15 mins

Total Time: 25 mins

Servings: 6

Yield: 6 servings

Ingredients

¼ cup olive oil

¼ cup sliced fresh mushrooms

¼ cup chopped onions

¼ cup chopped green bell peppers

6 eggs

¼ cup milk

¼ cup chopped fresh tomato

¼ cup shredded Cheddar cheese

Directions

Heat olive oil in a skillet or frying pan over medium-high heat. Add mushrooms, onions and peppers; saute until onions are transparent.

In a mixing bowl, beat together eggs and milk. Add egg mixture to vegetables; stir in tomatoes. Cook until eggs are set. When eggs are almost done, mix in cheese. Serve immediately.

Nutrition Facts (per serving)

182 Calories 16g Fat 2g Carbs 8g Protein

This grilled chicken marinade is the best! It is so flavorful and so simple to prep with easy pantry ingredients. Perfect for any occasion.

Prep Time: 10 mins

Cook Time: 10 mins

Additional Time: 4 hrs

Total Time: 4 hrs 20 mins

Servings: 5

Ingredients

¼ cup red wine vinegar

¼ cup reduced-sodium soy sauce

¼ cup olive oil

1 ½ teaspoons dried parsley flakes

½ teaspoon dried basil

½ teaspoon dried oregano

¼ teaspoon garlic powder

¼ teaspoon ground black pepper

5 skinless, boneless chicken breasts, thinly sliced

Directions

Gather all ingredients.

Whisk vinegar, soy sauce, olive oil, parsley, basil, oregano, garlic powder, and black pepper together in a bowl.

Pour into a resealable plastic bag. Add chicken, coat with the marinade, squeeze out excess air, and seal the bag. Marinate in the refrigerator, at least 4 hours.

Preheat grill for medium-low heat and lightly oil the grate. Drain and discard marinade.

Grill chicken on the preheated grill until no longer pink in the center, 4 to 5 minutes per side. An instant-read thermometer inserted into the center should read at least 165 degrees F (74 degrees C).

Editor's Note:

The nutrition data for this recipe includes the full amount of the marinade ingredients. The actual amount of the marinade consumed will vary.

Nutrition Facts (per serving)

233 Calories 14g Fat 2g Carbs 24g Protein

Rosemary Lemon Grilled Chicken

This simple, sensational marinade and sauce for grilled chicken is made with lemon, garlic, rosemary, and butter. Separate the marinade into thirds: 1/3 for marinating, 1/3 for basting, and 1/3 for topping.

Prep Time: 15 mins

Cook Time: 8 mins

Additional Time: 3 hrs

Total Time: 3 hrs 23 mins

Servings: 6

Ingredients

½ cup butter

½ cup fresh rosemary

3 cloves garlic

1 lemon, zested

¼ cup fresh lemon juice

6 (6 ounce) skinless, boneless chicken breast halves

salt and pepper to taste

Directions

In a food processor, blend butter, rosemary, garlic, lemon zest, and lemon juice together. Pour 1/3 of the blended mixture into a small bowl for marinade. Cover remaining mixture, and set aside.

Lightly season chicken breasts with salt and pepper. Rub chicken breasts with marinade. Place chicken breasts on a platter, cover, and refrigerate for 3 hours.

Preheat an outdoor grill for high heat and lightly oil the grate. Transfer half of the reserved rosemary and lemon mixture into a bowl for basting. Cover remaining mixture, and set aside for topping cooked chicken.

Cook chicken breasts on hot grill, basting with rosemary and lemon basting mixture, about 4 minutes per side. An instant-read thermometer inserted into the center should read at least 165 degrees F (74 degrees C). Remove chicken breasts from the grill, and top with remaining rosemary and lemon mixture.

Nutrition Facts (per serving)

331 Calories 18g Fat 2g Carbs 40g Protein

Tropical Grilled Chicken Breast

Living in South Florida, I get to enjoy a diverse culture, from all the Latin and Caribbean influence down here. Friends and family all enjoy this simple recipe, hope you do to . . .

Prep Time: 5 mins

Cook Time: 12 mins

Additional Time: 30 mins

Total Time: 47 mins

Servings: 4

Yield: 4 servings

Ingredients

½ cup orange juice

½ lime, juiced

1 tablespoon honey

1 teaspoon crushed red pepper flakes

4 (6 ounce) skinless, boneless chicken breast halves

1 tablespoon chopped fresh cilantro

Directions

Whisk together the orange juice, lime juice, honey, and red pepper flakes in a bowl, and pour into a resealable plastic bag. Add the chicken, coat with the marinade, squeeze out excess air, and seal the bag. Marinate in the refrigerator for 30 minutes.

Preheat an outdoor grill for medium-high heat, and lightly oil the grate.

Remove the chicken from the marinade, and shake off excess. Discard the remaining marinade. Place the chicken on the grill and cook the chicken breasts until no longer pink in the center and the juices run clear, about 6 to 8 minutes per side. An instant-read thermometer inserted into the center should read at least 165 degrees F (74 degrees C). Top with cilantro and serve.

Nutrition Facts (per serving)

223 Calories 4g Fat 9g Carbs 36g Protein

Learn how long to bake salmon at 400 degrees F with this easy recipe for delicious salmon fillets coated with Dijon-style mustard and seasoned bread crumbs drizzled with butter.

Prep Time: 10 mins

Cook Time: 15 mins

Total Time: 25 mins

Servings: 4

Ingredients

4 (4 ounce) fillets salmon

3 tablespoons prepared Dijon-style mustard

salt and ground black pepper to taste

¼ cup Italian-style dry bread crumbs

¼ cup butter, melted

Directions

Gather all ingredients. Preheat the oven to 400 degrees F (200 degrees C). Line a shallow baking pan with aluminum foil.

Place salmon fillets skin-side down on the prepared baking pan. Spread a thin layer of mustard on top of each fillet; season with salt and pepper.

Top with bread crumbs, then drizzle with melted butter.

Bake in the preheated oven until salmon flakes easily with a fork, about 15 minutes.

Serve and enjoy!

Breaded, baked salmon fillets topped with lemon slices, served alongside asparagus slices and rice pilaf on blue plates

Baked Salmon Fillets with Dijon Mustard. ALLRECIPES

Editor's Note:

Please note the slight difference in the recipe name, as well as differences in the ingredient amounts, cook times, and use of skinless salmon when using the magazine version of this recipe.

Nutrition Facts (per serving)

331 Calories 22g Fat 8g Carbs 25g Protein

Baked Salmon

This baked salmon is a great recipe for beginners. This was my first time making fish and it was a hit. Even my 9-year-old daughter who wouldn't ever dream of eating fish had half of my portion!

Prep Time: 15 mins

Cook Time: 35 mins

Additional Time: 1 hr

Total Time: 1 hr 50 mins

Servings: 2

Ingredients

6 tablespoons light olive oil

2 cloves garlic, minced

1 tablespoon lemon juice

1 tablespoon fresh parsley, chopped

1 teaspoon dried basil

1 teaspoon salt

1 teaspoon ground black pepper

2 (6 ounce) fillets salmon

Directions

Whisk olive oil, garlic, lemon juice, parsley, basil, salt, and pepper together in a medium bowl.

Arrange salmon fillets in a small glass or ceramic baking dish; pour marinade over salmon. Cover and marinate in the refrigerator for about 1 hour, turning occasionally.

Preheat the oven to 375 degrees F (190 degrees C).

Transfer salmon fillets onto a large piece of aluminum foil. Spoon marinade on top and fold up the foil to seal. Place sealed foil packs on a baking sheet.

Bake in preheated oven until fish flakes easily with a fork, about 35 to 45 minutes.

Serve hot and enjoy!

Editor's Note:

The nutrition data for this recipe includes information for the full amount of the marinade ingredients. Depending on marinating time, ingredients, cooking method, etc., the actual amount of the marinade consumed will vary.

Nutrition Facts (per serving)

613 Calories 52g Fat 3g Carbs 36g Protein

Many cooks are intimidated by cooking fresh fish and, as a result, miss out on the heart-healthy, brain-boosting, omega-3 fatty acids in salmon. Never fear, though — this recipe for baked salmon with coconut is foolproof!

Prep Time: 10 mins

Cook Time: 15 mins

Total Time: 25 mins

Servings: 4

Ingredients

4 (4 ounce) salmon fillets, skin removed

1 tablespoon lime or lemon juice

½ cup panko (Japanese bread crumbs, available in the Asian food aisle), or substitute dry bread crumbs

¼ cup flaked sweetened coconut

Salt and freshly ground pepper, to taste

Cooking spray

Directions

Preheat the oven to 425 degrees F (220 degrees C).

Place salmon fillets on a nonstick baking pan; brush juice on salmon.

In a shallow dish, combine panko, coconut, salt, and pepper. Dredge each salmon fillet in panko mixture and return to the baking pan. Spread leftover crumbs on top of each salmon fillet. Coat with cooking spray.

Bake in the preheated oven for 12 to 15 minutes. If desired, put under broiler until crust is golden brown.

Nutrition Facts (per serving)

264 Calories 14g Fat 12g Carbs 24g Protein

Yellow Squash and Tofu Stir Fry

A great, quick vegetarian dish that includes yellow squash, zucchini, and tofu, making for a beautifully-colored dish. Top with cheese, if desired. You can use butter instead of olive oil, if desired.

Prep Time: 20 mins

Cook Time: 15 mins

Total Time: 35 mins

Servings: 3

Yield: 3 servings

Ingredients

1 tablespoon olive oil, or as needed

3 cloves garlic, minced

1 yellow squash, cut into bite-size cubes

1 zucchini, cut into bite-size cubes

1 (12 ounce) package extra-firm tofu, cut into bite-size cubes

¼ cup brown sugar

3 tablespoons soy sauce

1 tablespoon sriracha sauce

salt and ground black pepper to taste

Directions

Heat olive oil in a large skillet or wok over medium-high heat. Cook and stir garlic in hot oil until just fragrant, about 30 seconds. Add squash and zucchini, cook and stir until vegetables soften, about 7 minutes. Transfer squash mixture to a bowl.

Place skillet back over medium-high heat, place tofu pieces in the skillet, and top with brown sugar and soy sauce. Cook and stir until each side of tofu is golden brown, 3 to 5 minutes.

Return squash mixture to the skillet; cook and stir until heated through, about 3 minutes. Stir in Sriracha sauce and season with salt and black pepper.

Nutrition Facts (per serving)

233 Calories 10g Fat 28g Carbs 12g Protein

When I get a craving for orange beef, I make up this tofu stir-fry! Pieces of firm tofu in a mildly spicy orange sauce. Serve over rice noodles, and use any vegetables you like!

Prep Time: 15 mins

Cook Time: 15 mins

Total Time: 30 mins

Servings: 4

Yield: 4 servings

Ingredients

¼ cup vegetable oil for frying

¼ cup cornstarch

1 (16 ounce) package firm tofu, drained and cut into strips

2 tablespoons soy sauce

½ cup orange juice

¼ cup warm water

1 tablespoon sugar

1 teaspoon chili paste

1 teaspoon cornstarch

1 tablespoon vegetable oil

2 carrots, sliced

Directions

Heat 1/4 cup oil in a wok over medium-high heat. Place the 1/4 cup cornstarch in a dish; press tofu slices in the cornstarch to coat on all sides. Stir-fry in the wok 5 minutes, or until golden brown on all sides. Drain tofu on paper towels. Allow wok to cool, and wipe clean.

In a bowl, mix the soy sauce, orange juice, water, sugar, chili paste, and cornstarch until smooth.

Heat the remaining 1 tablespoon oil in the wok, and stir-fry the carrots until tender. Form a well in the center of the carrots, and pour in the sauce. Bring sauce to a boil. Mix tofu into the wok, and continue cooking until coated with the sauce.

Note

We have determined the nutritional value of oil for frying based on a retention value of 10% after cooking. The exact amount may vary depending on cook time and temperature, ingredient density, and the specific type of oil used.

Nutrition Facts (per serving)

286 Calories 15g Fat 23g Carbs 19g Protein

A very tasty, hearty, easy to prepare soup that also freezes well.

Ingredients

1 pound lean ground beef

1 ½ cups dry lentils, rinsed

1 cup chopped carrots

1 cup chopped onion

1 cup chopped celery

3 cups water

1 teaspoon salt

ground black pepper to taste

2 cubes beef bouillon cube

6 cups tomato-vegetable juice cocktail

1 (4.5 ounce) can mushrooms, drained

1 dash Worcestershire sauce

Directions

Brown beef; break meat into small pieces while cooking. Drain.

Place meat in a big pot with lid. Add lentils, vegetables, water, salt, pepper, bouillon, vegetable juice, mushrooms, and Worcestershire sauce. Cook on high until it boils. Reduce heat to low, and cover. Simmer for about 1 1/2 to 2 hours, or until lentils are tender. Stir occasionally.

Nutrition Facts (per serving)

385 Calories 14g Fat 39g Carbs 25g Protein

Winter Lentil Vegetable Soup

This soup has very little fat, is cheap and easy to make and delicious. Our family practically lives on it in the winter and I usually double the recipe. Sprinkle grated cheddar on top if you wish. If you can't hang around long enough for this to cook, put it in a slow cooker.

Prep Time: 20 mins

Cook Time: 1 hr 30 mins

Additional Time: 1 hr 10 mins

Total Time: 3 hrs

Servings: 6

Yield: 6 to 1 - cup servings

Ingredients

½ cup red or green lentils

1 cup chopped onion

1 stalk celery, chopped

2 cups shredded cabbage

1 (28 ounce) can whole peeled tomatoes, chopped

2 cups chicken broth

3 carrots, chopped

1 clove garlic, crushed

1 teaspoon salt

½ teaspoon ground black pepper

¼ teaspoon white sugar

½ teaspoon dried basil

½ teaspoon dried thyme

¼ teaspoon curry powder

Directions

Place the lentils into a stockpot or a Dutch oven and add water to twice the depth of the lentils. Bring to a boil, then lower heat and let simmer for about 15 minutes. Drain and rinse lentils; return them to the pot.

Add onion, celery, cabbage, tomatoes, chicken broth, carrots and garlic to the pot and season with salt, pepper, sugar, basil, thyme and curry. Cook, simmering for 1 1/2 to 2 hours or until desired tenderness is achieved.

Cook's Note:

Combine ingredients in a slow cooker and cook on Low for 8 to 10 hours, or on High for about 4 hours, or until lentils have broken down and vegetables are tender.

Easy Cleanup

Try using a liner in your slow cooker for easier cleanup.

Nutrition Facts (per serving)

112 Calories 1g Fat 22g Carbs 6g Protein

Instant Pot Lentil Vegetable Soup

Warm and healthy one-pot dish cooked in an Instant Pot.

Prep Time: 20 mins

Cook Time: 40 mins

Additional Time: 5 mins

Total Time: 1 hr 5 mins

Servings: 8

Ingredients

1 teaspoon vegetable oil

1 large onion, chopped

1 red bell pepper, chopped

1 carrot, chopped

3 cloves garlic, minced

4 (14.5 ounce) cans chicken broth

1 pound lentils, rinsed and drained

2 medium zucchini, chopped

1 small eggplant, peeled and chopped

1 (14 ounce) can diced tomatoes with juice

1 tablespoon dried parsley

2 teaspoons ground cumin

1 teaspoon salt

2 teaspoons lemon zest

1 tablespoon lemon juice

Directions

Place oil in a multi-functional pressure cooker (such as Instant Pot) and select Saute function. Add onion, bell pepper, and carrot; cook and stir until the onion has softened and turned translucent, about 5 minutes. Stir in garlic and saute until fragrant, about 1 minute. Cancel Saute function.

Add chicken broth, lentils, zucchini, eggplant, diced tomatoes with juice, parsley, cumin, and salt to the pot. Close and lock the lid. Select high pressure according to manufacturer's instructions; set timer for 20 minutes. Allow 10 to 15 minutes for pressure to build.

Release pressure carefully using the quick-release method according to manufacturer's instructions, about 5 minutes. Unlock and remove the lid. Stir in lemon juice and zest.

Tips

To make this vegetarian, use vegetable broth in place of chicken broth.

Nutrition Facts (per serving)

268 Calories

2g Fat

45g Carbs

18g Protein

This quinoa salad light and citrusy, easy to make for a great summer meal, and a great new way to enjoy quinoa. Lime juice and cilantro give a refreshing kick, while quinoa and black beans make it hearty and filling.

Prep Time: 20 mins

Cook Time: 15 mins

Total Time: 35 mins

Servings: 6

How to Store Quinoa Salad

Store the quinoa salad in an airtight container in the refrigerator for about five days.

Can You Freeze Quinoa Salad?

Yes! You can freeze the quinoa salad for up to six months. Thaw the salad in the refrigerator overnight.

Ingredients

2 cups water

1 cup quinoa

¼ cup extra-virgin olive oil

2 limes, juiced

2 teaspoons ground cumin

1 teaspoon salt

½ teaspoon red pepper flakes, or more to taste

1 ½ cups halved cherry tomatoes

1 (15 ounce) can black beans, drained and rinsed

5 green onions, finely chopped

¼ cup chopped fresh cilantro

salt and ground black pepper to taste

Directions

Bring water and quinoa to a boil in a saucepan. Reduce heat to medium-low, cover, and simmer until quinoa is tender and water has been absorbed, 10 to 15 minutes. Set aside to cool.

Meanwhile, whisk olive oil, lime juice, cumin, salt, and red pepper flakes together in a small bowl.

Combine quinoa, tomatoes, black beans, and green onions in a large bowl. Pour dressing over quinoa mixture; toss to coat. Stir in cilantro; season with salt and black pepper.

Serve immediately or chill salad in the refrigerator.

Nutrition Facts (per serving)

270 Calories 12g Fat 34g Carbs 9g Protein

This Greek quinoa salad is one of my absolute favorite recipes. It's so flavorful and always a big hit with my family and friends. Trust me, you'll want to eat every single bite!

Prep Time: 15 mins

Cook Time: 15 mins

Additional Time: 1 hr 10 mins

Total Time: 1 hr 40 mins

Servings: 10

Ingredients

3 ½ cups chicken broth

2 cups quinoa

1 cup halved grape tomatoes

¾ cup chopped fresh parsley

½ cup sliced pitted kalamata olives

½ cup minced red onion

4 ounces chopped feta cheese, or more to taste

3 tablespoons olive oil

3 tablespoons red wine vinegar

2 cloves garlic, minced

1 lemon, halved

salt and ground black pepper to taste

Directions

Bring broth and quinoa to a boil in a saucepan. Reduce heat to medium-low, cover, and simmer until quinoa is tender and water has been absorbed, 15 to 20 minutes. Transfer quinoa to a large bowl and set aside to cool, about 10 minutes.

Mix tomatoes, parsley, kalamata olives, onion, feta cheese, olive oil, vinegar, and garlic into quinoa. Squeeze lemon juice over quinoa salad, season with salt and pepper, and toss to coat. Chill in refrigerator, 1 to 4 hours.

Nutrition Facts (per serving)

227 Calories 11g Fat 26g Carbs 7g Protein

An easy Mediterranean quinoa salad that's lovely and light with bright lemon and fresh herb flavors. This salad is equally good warm or cold.

Prep Time: 15 mins

Cook Time: 15 mins

Total Time: 30 mins

Servings: 8

Yield: 4 cups

Ingredients

2 cups water

2 cubes chicken bouillon

1 clove garlic, smashed

1 cup uncooked quinoa

2 large cooked chicken breasts - cut into bite size pieces (Optional)

1 large red onion, diced

1 large green bell pepper, diced

½ cup chopped kalamata olives

½ cup crumbled feta cheese

¼ cup chopped fresh parsley

¼ cup chopped fresh chives

½ teaspoon salt

⅔ cup fresh lemon juice

1 tablespoon balsamic vinegar

¼ cup olive oil

Directions

Bring water, bouillon cubes, and garlic to a boil in a saucepan. Stir in quinoa; reduce heat to medium-low, cover, and simmer until quinoa is tender and water has been absorbed, 15 to 20 minutes. Discard garlic clove and transfer quinoa into a large bowl.

Add chicken, onion, bell pepper, olives, feta cheese, parsley, chives, and salt to quinoa; drizzle lemon juice, balsamic vinegar, and olive oil on top. Stir until evenly mixed. Serve warm or refrigerate and serve cold.

Nutrition Facts (per serving)

278 Calories 14g Fat 20g Carbs 18g Protein

Perfect Ten Baked Cod

This baked cod recipe is simple, fast, and delicious. The fish is baked in butter, then topped with lemon juice, white wine, and buttery crackers for the perfect ten dinner. This dish is a favorite of ours from a local restaurant. Serve with rice pilaf and sautéed spinach with garlic. Yummy!

Prep Time: 10 mins

Cook Time: 25 mins

Total Time: 35 mins

Servings: 4

Yield: 4 servings

Cod Loins vs. Cod Fillets

Cod loin, considered the prime cut for cod, is cut from the middle section, or the thickest part of the fillet. When cooked, it's generally more moist and succulent, and cooks more evenly than standard cod fillets. Cod loins are also sold as smaller cuts, which makes them easier to work with. Cod fillets on the other hand are vertical cuts from the body, and can often be too big for a single portion. You can substitute cod fillets for loins in this recipe, just be sure to adjust the cooking time if your fillet is large.

What Is the Best Wine to Use?

We recommend a light, dry white wine like Sauvignon Blanc, Pinot Grigio, or an unoaked

Chardonnay. These will bring out the dish's flavor without overwhelming it. Avoid rich, oaky white wines like an oaky Chardonnay. And no need to splurge on a fancy wine — as wine cooks, the subtle nuances of a more expensive wine will be lost.

Ingredients

4 tablespoons butter, divided

½ sleeve buttery round crackers (such as Ritz®), crushed

1 pound thick-cut cod loin

½ medium lemon, juiced

¼ cup dry white wine

1 tablespoon chopped fresh parsley

1 tablespoon chopped green onion

1 medium lemon, cut into wedges

Directions

Gather all ingredients.

Preheat the oven to 400 degrees F (200 degrees C).

Place 2 tablespoons butter in a microwave-safe bowl. Melt in the microwave on high, about 30 seconds. Stir buttery round crackers into melted butter.

Place remaining 2 tablespoons butter in a 7x11-inch baking dish. Melt in the preheated oven, 1 to 3 minutes. Remove dish from oven.

Coat both sides of cod in melted butter in the baking dish.

Bake cod in the preheated oven for 10 minutes. Remove from oven; top with lemon juice, wine, and cracker mixture. Return to the oven and bake until fish is opaque and flakes easily with a fork, about 10 more minutes.

Garnish with parsley and green onion and serve with lemon wedges.

Nutrition Facts (per serving)

280 Calories 16g Fat 9g Carbs 21g Protein

Baked Cod with Boursin Herb Cheese

Use Boursin or Allouette Cheese and canned tomatoes seasoned with onion, peppers and garlic to make this dish with fresh cod. It's an outstanding fish recipe for a quick and easy-to-prepare dinner. Add a tossed salad, a green vegetable side dish, and your dinner is complete. Olive oil may be substituted for the butter.

Prep Time: 15 mins

Cook Time: 25 mins

Total Time: 40 mins

Servings: 4

Yield: 4 servings

Ingredients

2 tablespoons butter, melted

2 pounds fresh cod fillets

1 (4 ounce) package Boursin cheese with herbs, room temperature

1 (14.5 ounce) can diced tomatoes with garlic, onion, and peppers, drained

salt and ground black pepper to taste

2 tablespoons shredded Parmesan cheese

Directions

Preheat oven to 400 degrees F (200 degrees C).

Pour 1 tablespoon melted butter into baking dish to coat bottom. Arrange the cod fillets in the dish. Pat fillets dry using a paper towel. Spread the Boursin cheese evenly over the fillets. Pour the tomatoes over the tops. Season with salt and pepper to taste. Sprinkle with Parmesan cheese. Drizzle with remaining 1 tablespoon butter.

Bake, uncovered, in preheated oven for 25 minutes.

Nutrition Facts (per serving)

394 Calories 21g Fat 8g Carbs 45g Protein

A healthier adaptation of a Pad Thai recipe. Serve with extra lime wedges.

Prep Time: 45 mins

Cook Time: 12 mins

Total Time: 57 mins

Servings: 4

Yield: 4 servings

Ingredients

3 large zucchini

¼ cup chicken stock

2 ½ tablespoons tamarind paste

2 tablespoons low-sodium soy sauce

2 tablespoons oyster sauce

1 ½ tablespoons Asian chile pepper sauce

1 tablespoon Worcestershire sauce

1 tablespoon fresh lime juice

1 tablespoon white sugar

2 tablespoons sesame oil

1 tablespoon chopped garlic

12 ounces skinless, boneless chicken breasts, cut into 1-inch cubes

8 ounces peeled and deveined shrimp

2 eggs, beaten

2 tablespoons water, or as needed (Optional)

3 cups bean sprouts, divided

6 green onions, chopped into 1-inch pieces

2 tablespoons chopped unsalted dry-roasted peanuts

¼ cup chopped fresh basil

Directions

Make zucchini noodles using a spiralizer.

Whisk chicken stock, tamarind paste, soy sauce, oyster sauce, chile pepper sauce, Worcestershire sauce, lime juice, and sugar together in a small bowl to make a smooth sauce.

Heat sesame oil in a wok or large skillet over high heat. Add garlic and stir until fragrant, about 10 seconds. Add chicken and shrimp; cook and stir until chicken is no longer pink in the center and the juices run clear, 5 to 7 minutes.

Push chicken and shrimp to the sides of the wok to make a space in the center. Pour eggs and scramble until firm, 2 to 3 minutes. Add zucchini noodles and sauce; cook and stir, adding water if needed, about 3 minutes. Add 2 cups bean sprouts and green onions; cook and stir until combined, 1 to 2 minutes.

Remove wok from heat and sprinkle peanuts over noodles. Serve garnished with remaining 1 cup bean sprouts and fresh basil.

Nutrition Facts (per serving)

370 Calories 15g Fat 28g Carbs 36g Protein

Spicy Grilled Shrimp

This grilled shrimp recipe is fast and easy to prepare and destined to be the hit of any barbeque. And, weather not permitting, the shrimp cook up great under the broiler, too.

Prep Time: 15 mins

Cook Time: 5 mins

Total Time: 20 mins

Servings: 6

How to Store Grilled Shrimp Leftovers

Store your grilled shrimp leftovers in an airtight container in the refrigerator for up to three days. Put them to good use by tossing them in one of our favorite Shrimp Salads.

Ingredients

1 large clove garlic

1 teaspoon coarse salt

1 teaspoon paprika

½ teaspoon cayenne pepper

2 tablespoons olive oil

2 teaspoons lemon juice

2 pounds large shrimp, peeled and deveined

8 wedges lemon, for garnish

Directions

Gather the ingredients. Preheat a grill for medium heat.

Crush garlic and salt together in a small bowl with a fork.

Mix in paprika and cayenne. Stir in olive oil and lemon juice to form a paste.

Combine garlic paste and shrimp in a large bowl and toss until shrimp are evenly coated.

Lightly oil the grill grate. Grill shrimp until opaque, 2 to 3 minutes per side.

Transfer to a serving dish, garnish with lemon wedges, and serve.

Editor's Note:

The salt amount has been reduced based on review feedback. The original recipe called for 1 tablespoon.

Nutrition Facts (per serving)

164 Calories

6g Fat

3g Carbs

25g Protein

Conclusion

A sugar-free diet (or no-sugar diet) is a diet that excludes added sugars and most processed foods. This type of diet is similar to a low-glycemic index diet and low-carb diet in that it helps reduce your body's reliance on glucose (sugar) for energy.

Benefits of a sugar-free diet include weight loss, helping normalize blood sugar, preventing insulin resistance, reducing cravings, giving you more energy and keeping you feeling fuller for longer after eating.

To reduce the amount of sugar in your diet, try focusing on making some of the following changes: Reduce or avoid sugary foods like cookies, cakes, candy and soft drinks; pair carbohydrates with proteins and healthy fats to make your meals more satisfying; consume unprocessed complex carbs instead of simple carbs; lower your intake of flour and white refined grains; eat more high-fiber foods like veggies, beans, legumes, nuts and seeds; and eat smaller amounts of starchy foods like white potatoes, white bread, rice, etc.

Reducing or eliminating added sugar from your diet can lead to improved health outcomes by reducing your chance of health issues such as diabetes, heart disease, and obesity.

Whether you choose to follow it for a short period or as a long-term lifestyle choice, consulting with a healthcare provider or dietitian is crucial to ensure it aligns with your individual health goals. Prioritizing whole, unprocessed foods and making mindful choices in your diet can pave the way to a healthier and sugar-smart future.